Affirmations For a Health Pregnancy

To help you manage fears, find balance
and affirm your loving connection
to your baby

Andreia Trigo

ISBN 10: 197786192X
ISBN 13: 978-1977861924

This book is dedicated to my dear family, who have offered me their unyielding support, helped me mourn the losses and ultimately rise above the challenges of infertility.

*

Each fertility journey is unique and challenging in its own way. And every mother has times when she feels afraid or has doubts in her pregnancy. This is completely normal. Affirmations are a way of managing those emotions and doubts, finding balance and creating an amazing connection with your own body and with your baby.

What is an affirmation?

An affirmation is a declaration or a strong statement of something that is true. When repeated daily, over time, the intention of the positive outcome becomes an internalised belief. When we believe without a doubt that something is true, we are increasing the likelihood of what we want to manifest actually happening.
The way you think about yourself, your body, your baby and pregnancy itself have an impact on you, on your relationship with yourself and with others who are meaningful to you.

So, next time you feel fear or stress, take a deep breath and read an affirmation out loud. Repeat it 3 times. Allow it to enter your mind, body and soul and become part of you.
Some of the affirmations in this book might resonate with you more than others. Choose the ones that are meaningful to you.

You are doing amazing in your fertility journey!

Andreia Trigo

Table of Contents

1.

Getting Ready

I am ready to become pregnant.
I now release anything that is
holding me back from becoming
pregnant.

I take care of myself and prepare my body for a healthy pregnancy.

I relax and I easily become
pregnant.

I now release all emotional blocks that prevent me from conceiving a baby.

I release fears about age and time.

I let go of the need to control when I become pregnant. I trust that I will become pregnant at exactly the right time.

I trust my body. My body knows
exactly what to do to conceive a
healthy baby.

I have everything it takes right now
to become pregnant.

I allow myself to be loved, and to create a new life out of that love.

I willingly release old thinking patterns based on fear and self-doubt. I allow new ones based on love and self-confidence.

My eggs are healthy and happy to
be release during my next ovulation.

I allow new beginnings in my life.

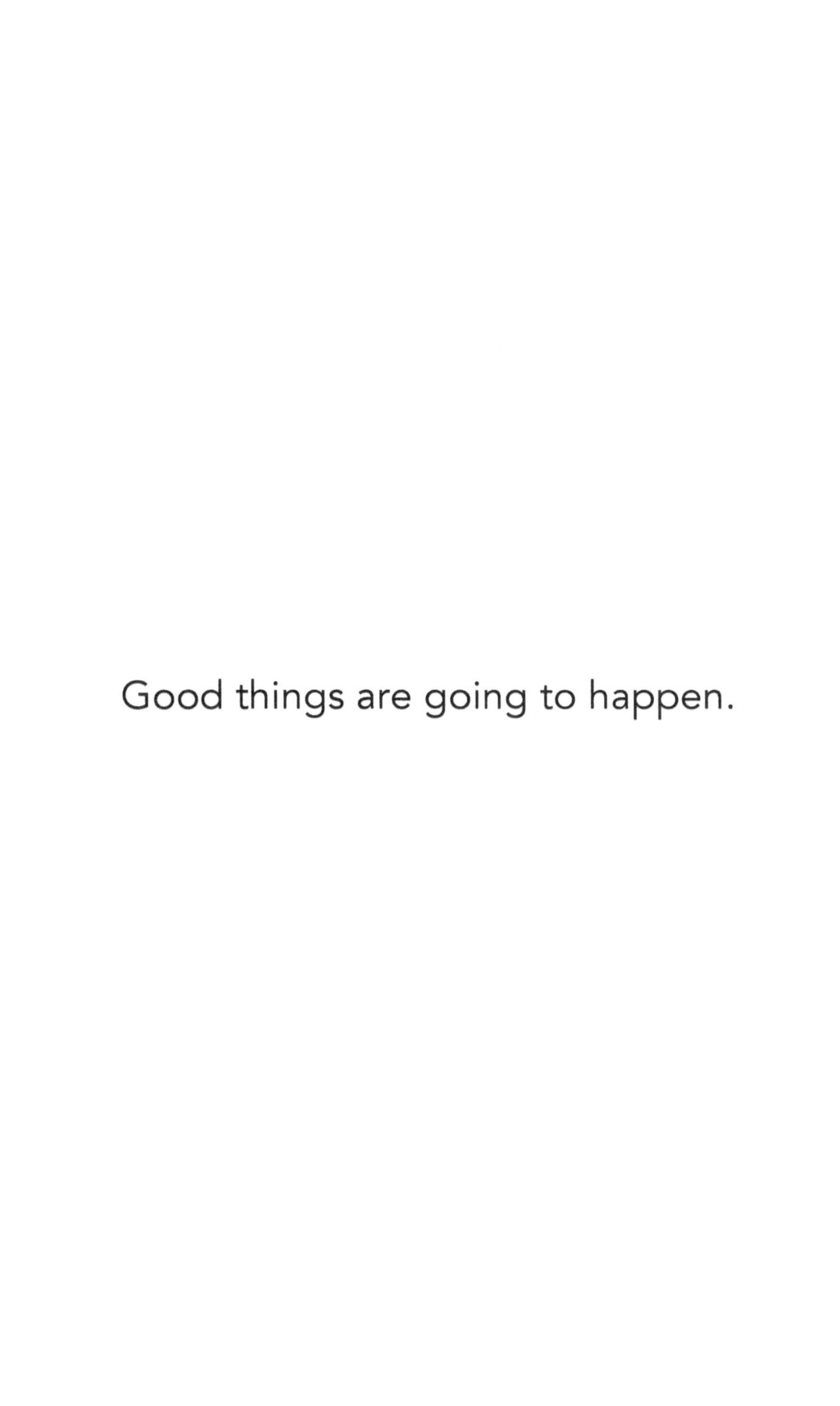

Good things are going to happen.

I accept the gift of life within myself.

I trust that the universe gives me exactly what I need at exactly the right time. Everything works out perfectly.

I accept the responsibilities of motherhood and I know I will rise to the occasion when the time comes.

I now release all unwanted built-up emotional patterns that prevent me from connecting to my inner self.

My courage is stronger than
my fear.

The most perfect egg is preparing to be released by my ovary and the most perfect sperm is preparing to fertilize it.

2.

My Baby and Pregnancy

This pregnancy and baby are special
and meant to be.

My baby is nestled safely in
my womb.

I am excited to meet this baby while
also being calm and patient
through today.

Everything I feel and experience is part of the great lesson of motherhood.

My baby is growing and developing
just as it should.

I am grateful to be able to feel a life growing inside of me.

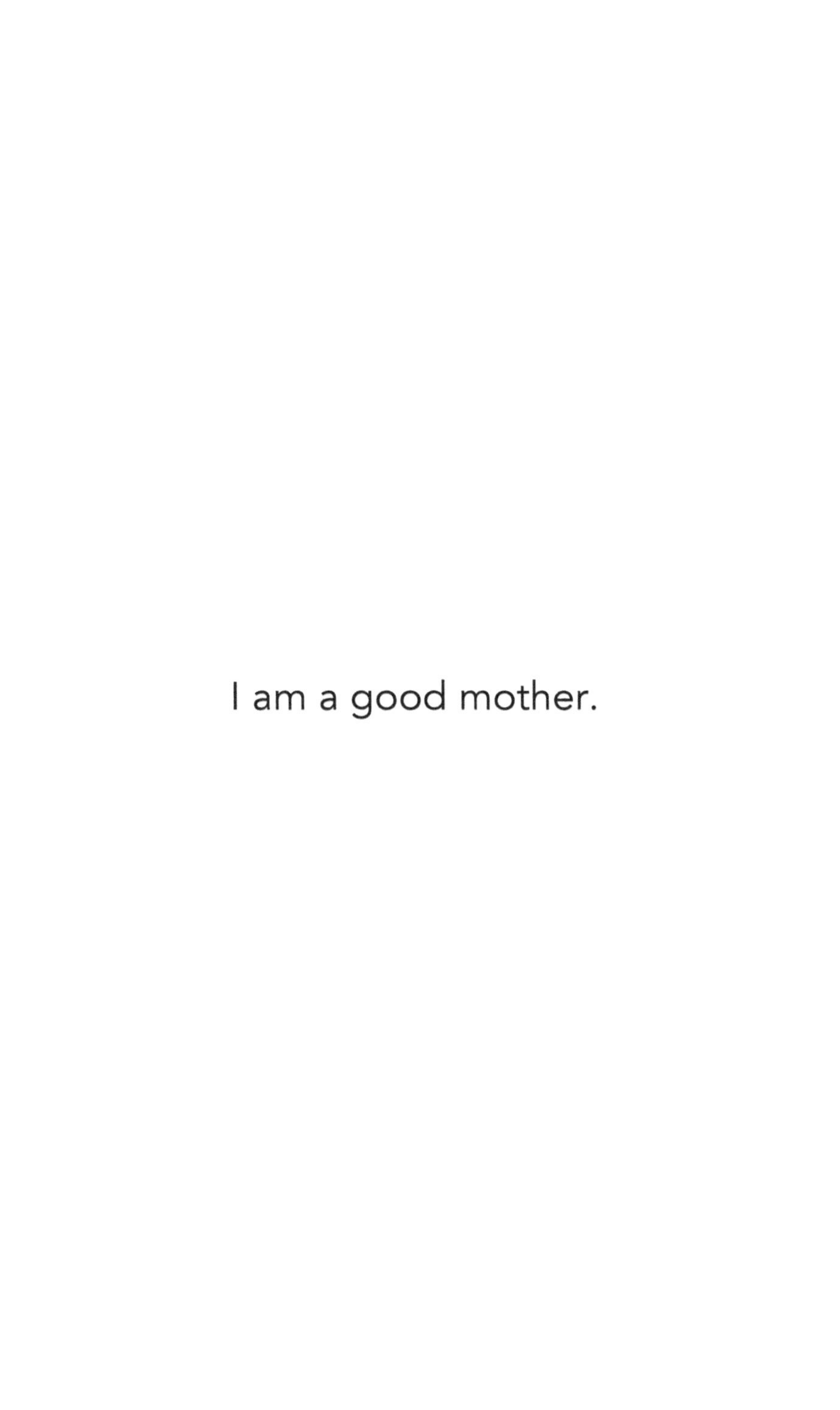

I am a good mother.

My life is important,
so is my baby's.

My baby feels my love for him//her.

My baby is a miracle and I
appreciate this opportunity to learn
to become a mother.

My pregnancy is perfect. I am delivering a happy, healthy baby.

I am in perfect health. My baby is in perfect health. This pregnancy comes to a perfect end.

My baby will be born at the
perfect time.

As my healthy baby grows within
me, I am more attuned than ever to
the perfect rhythms of nature and
my own body.

Each pregnancy is a unique and
beautiful experience.
I am consciously enjoying this
unique journey.

My choices throughout this pregnancy are based on facts not fear.

I conceived a beautiful baby and I
am delivering a beautiful child.

My love and connection with this child within me humbles me every day. I am blessed and I know it.

I conceived this baby in love. I am delivering this baby in love. I will raise this baby with love.

My baby is coming to meet me at exactly the right time, in exactly the right way. I got this.

I trust my baby to choose their perfect birthday, and I wait patiently and calmly for their arrival.

Me and my baby are one. I now choose to create peace within me and around me.

I am the most important person in
my baby's world. How I feel matters
and I choose to feel safe.

I choose to believe good things about pregnancy, birth and motherhood.

3.

My Body and Mind

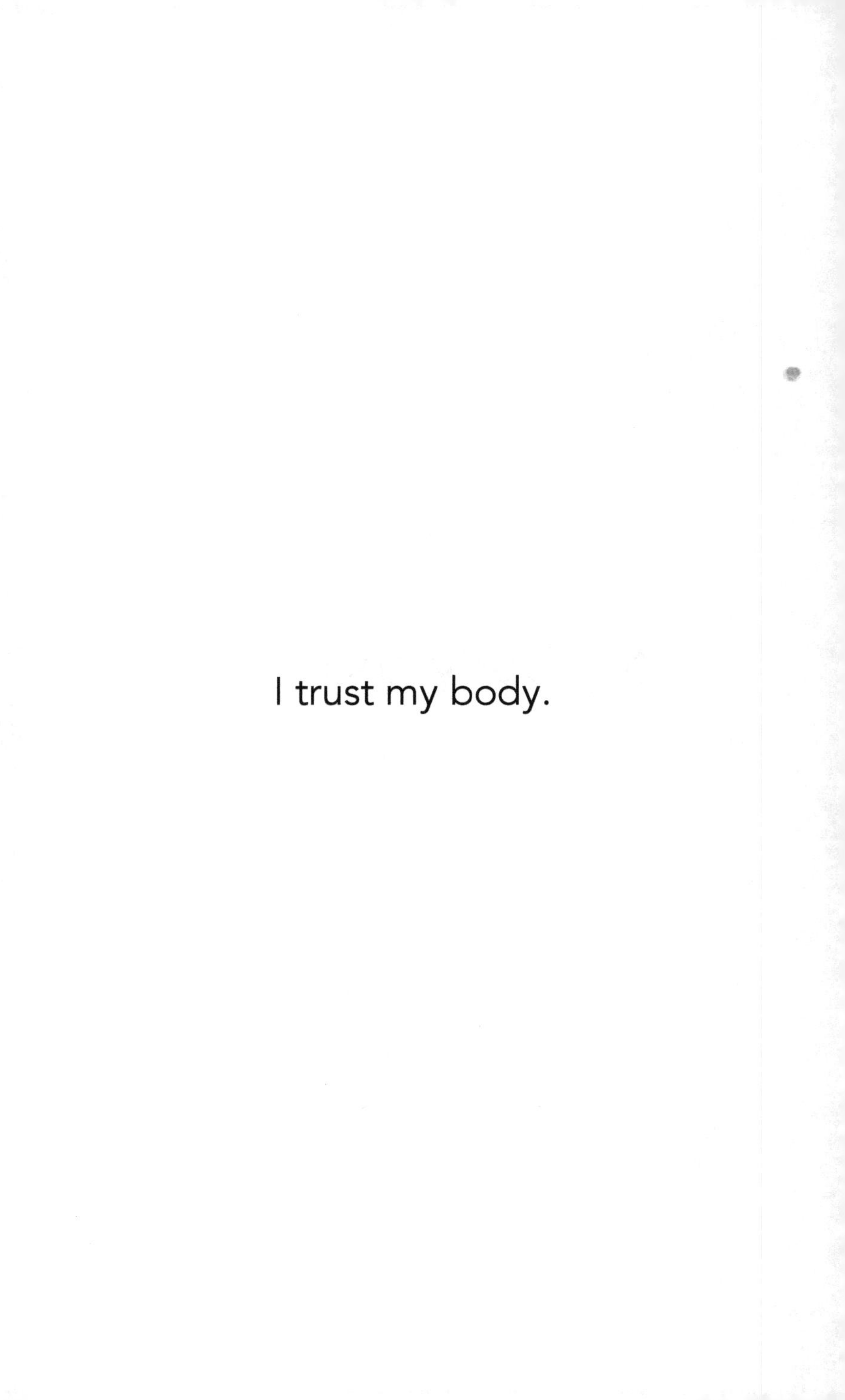

I trust my body.

New balance is coming to my body.

My body knows how to conceive a
healthy baby.

My reproductive organs work in
perfect harmony with my body to
allow an easy conception.

I surrender to the power of nature
as I celebrate a new cycle of birth
within myself.

My body is beautiful just the
way it is.

I love my pregnant body.

I am calm and centered when looking forward to the birth of my baby.

I accept the help of others with an open heart and mind.

I have the confidence to ask for help
and receive help when I need it.

I am listening to my body and
its needs.

I trust my body to work efficiently during pregnancy, labor, birth and breastfeeding.

I am an amazing mother about to
have an amazing baby.

I am strong and healthy and sailing right through this pregnancy.

I choose to see the beauty in this whole process of bringing a new life into the world.

I am calm, cool and confident
throughout my pregnancy. This is
the most beautiful nine months
of my life.

There may be difficult days during
this pregnancy, but I am strong,
determined and resilient.

As my healthy baby grows within me, I am more attuned than ever to the perfect rhythms of nature and my own body.

My body is beautifully nourishing
the child I carry. My child is
perfectly healthy.

My choices throughout this pregnancy are based on facts not fear.

I am highly-capable mother-to-be. If there are hard decisions to make, I can and I will make them.

Breathing in, I know I am a great mother. Breathing out, I AM a great mother.

I now release all unwanted built-up emotional patterns that prevent me from connecting to my inner self.

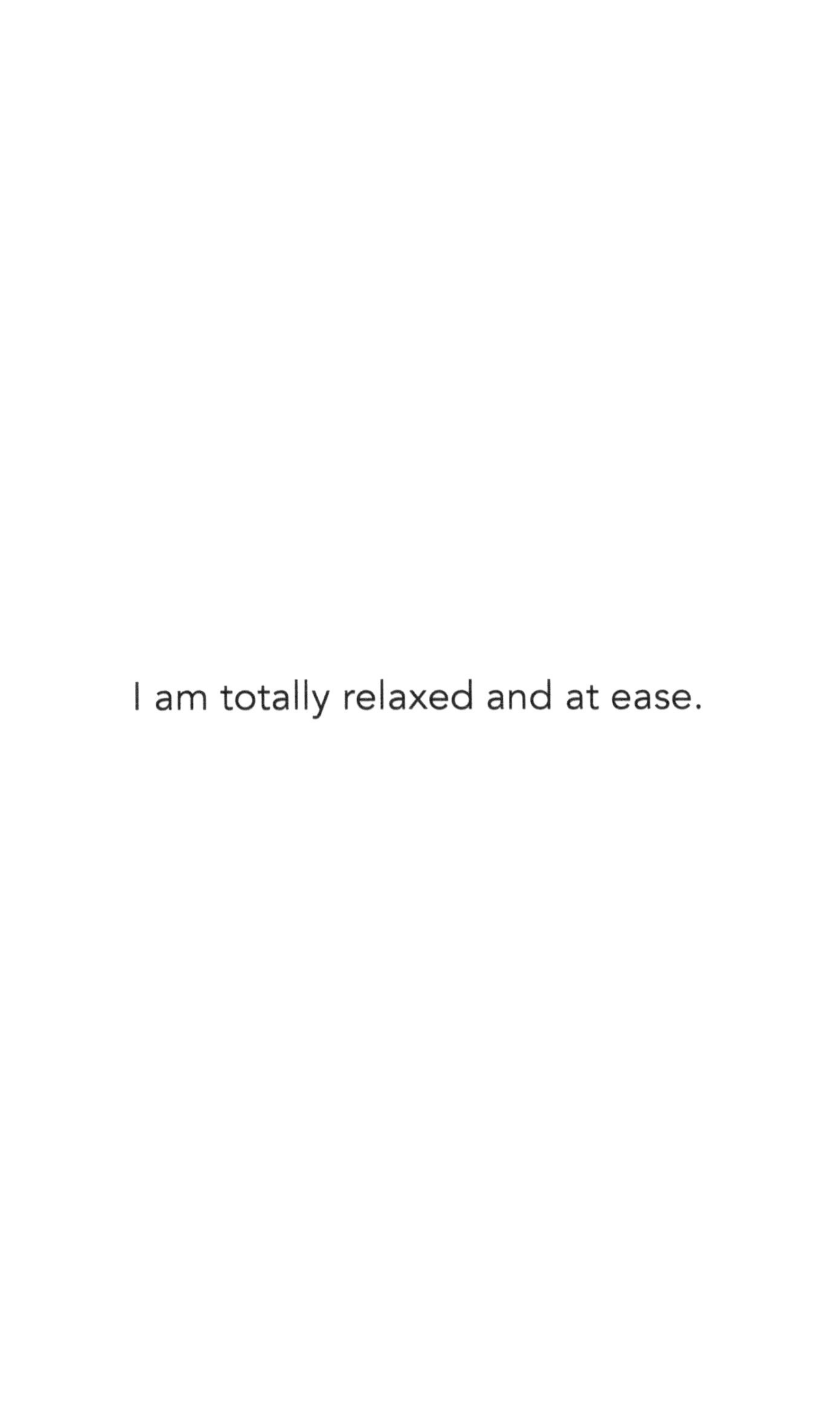

I am totally relaxed and at ease.

I am becoming more and more confident about my ability to have a child.

My sadness lifts away and renewed sense of hope settles in my heart.

I will not obsess over things that are
out of my control.

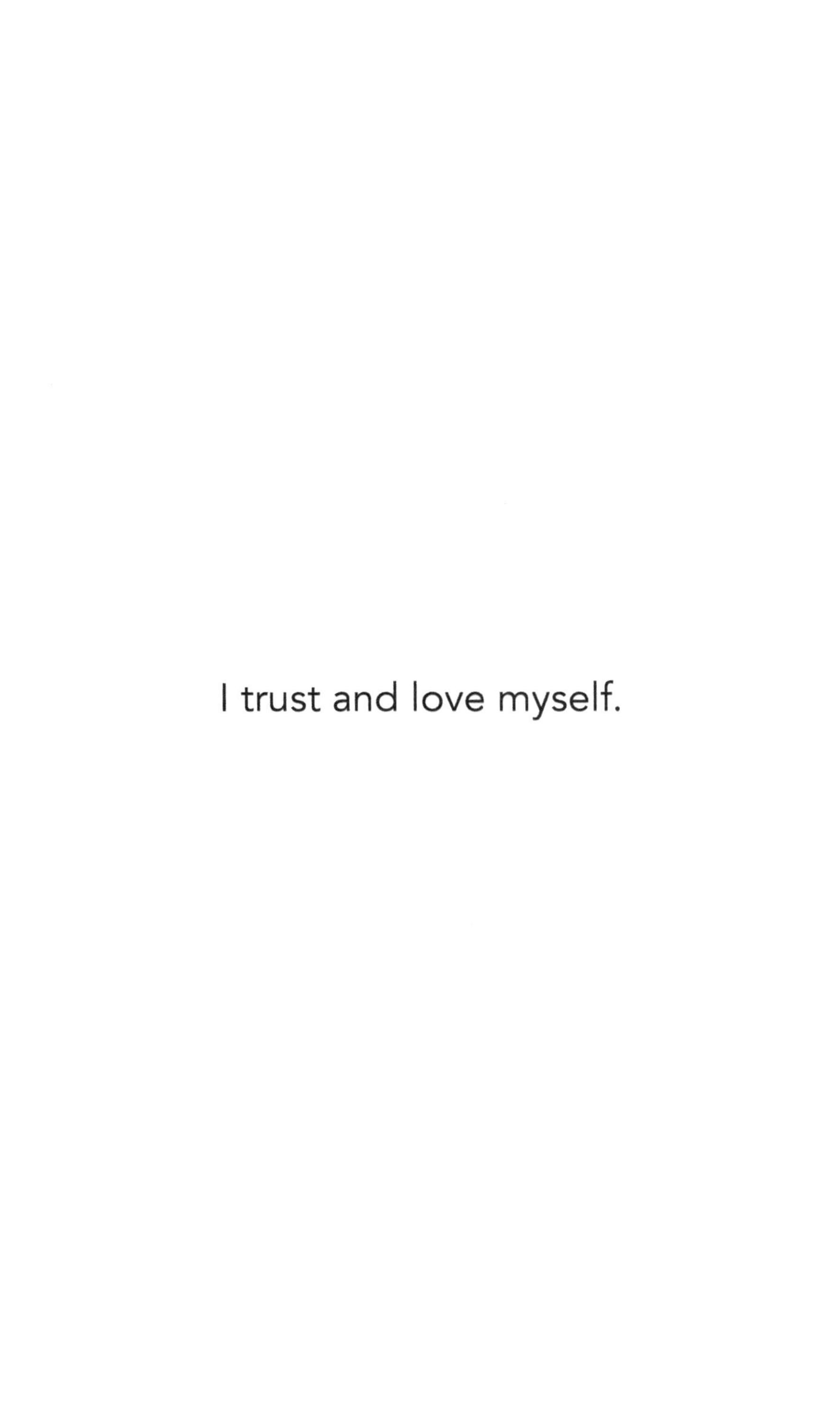

I trust and love myself.

I am too positive to be doubtful, too optimistic to be fearful, and too determined to be defeated.

4.

My Habits

I choose a healthy lifestyle that enhances my fertility.

I choose healthy foods every day. I now crave only foods that increase my wellbeing.

I easily avoid hydrogenated, highly processed foods and I enjoy simple foods made by nature.

The foods I am eating are nourishing me and my baby.

I take care of myself and prepare my body for a healthy pregnancy.

I'm listening to my body and
its needs.

I am absolutely committed to providing my child with a safe and happy home environment.

As the motherhood chapter of my life begins, I am ready to make it a beautiful chapter in my life.

I visualize myself after a perfect delivery. I am home loving and playing with my beautiful baby.

I am a great mother. My new baby
is lucky to have me.

I walk into every situation
expecting the best.

I now choose positive thoughts that nurture and support my life.

My courage is stronger than
my fear.

Nothing is important enough
to stress me.

5.

My Partner and
Support Network

I am loving and thankful toward my partner, who is supportive through my pregnancy.

I am surrounded by love and my baby feels this.

I am worthy of love and have the
capacity to love.

I have an amazing support system.

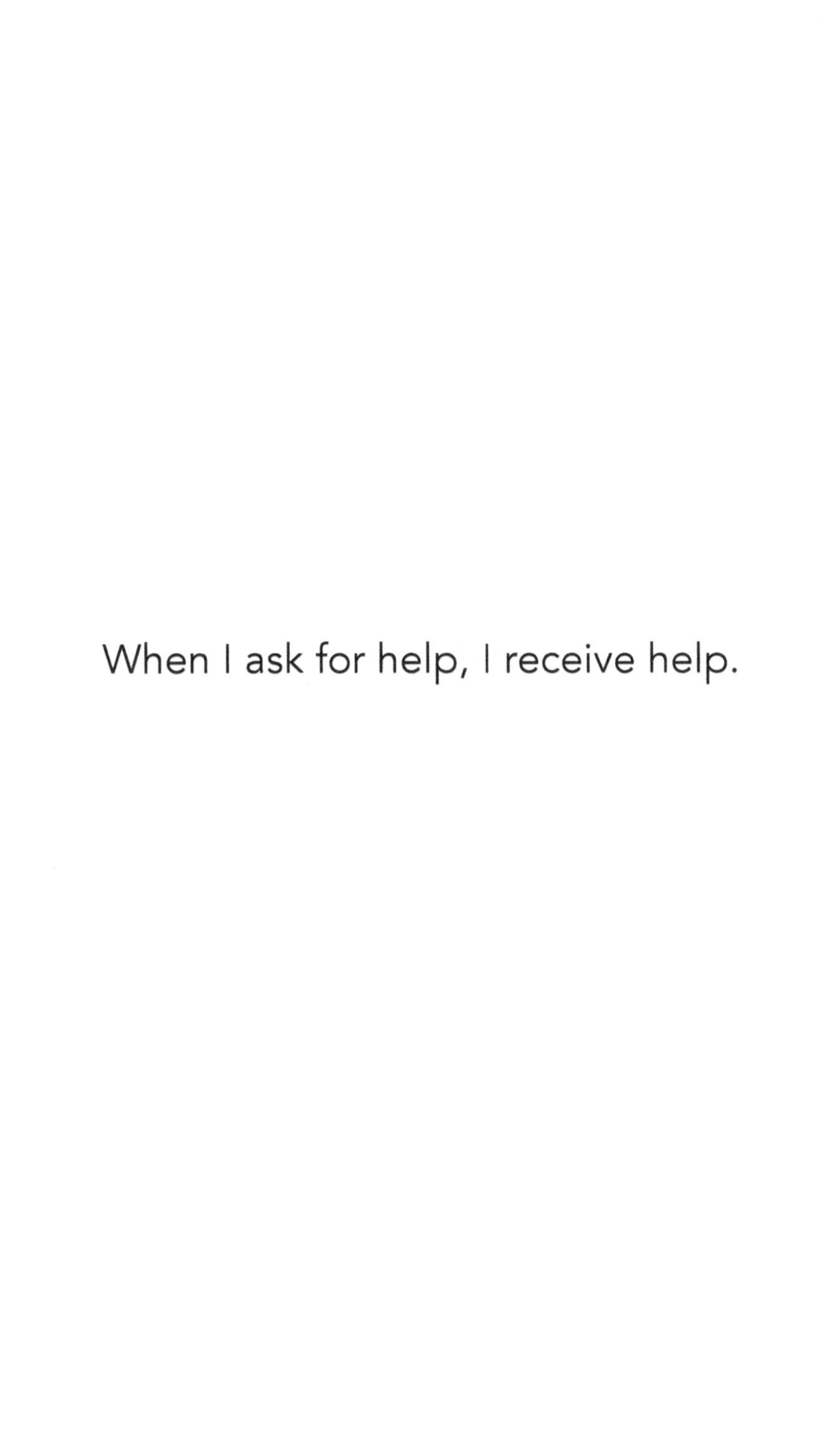

When I ask for help, I receive help.

My doctor and I are on the same
page. We are partners in delivering
a healthy, happy baby.